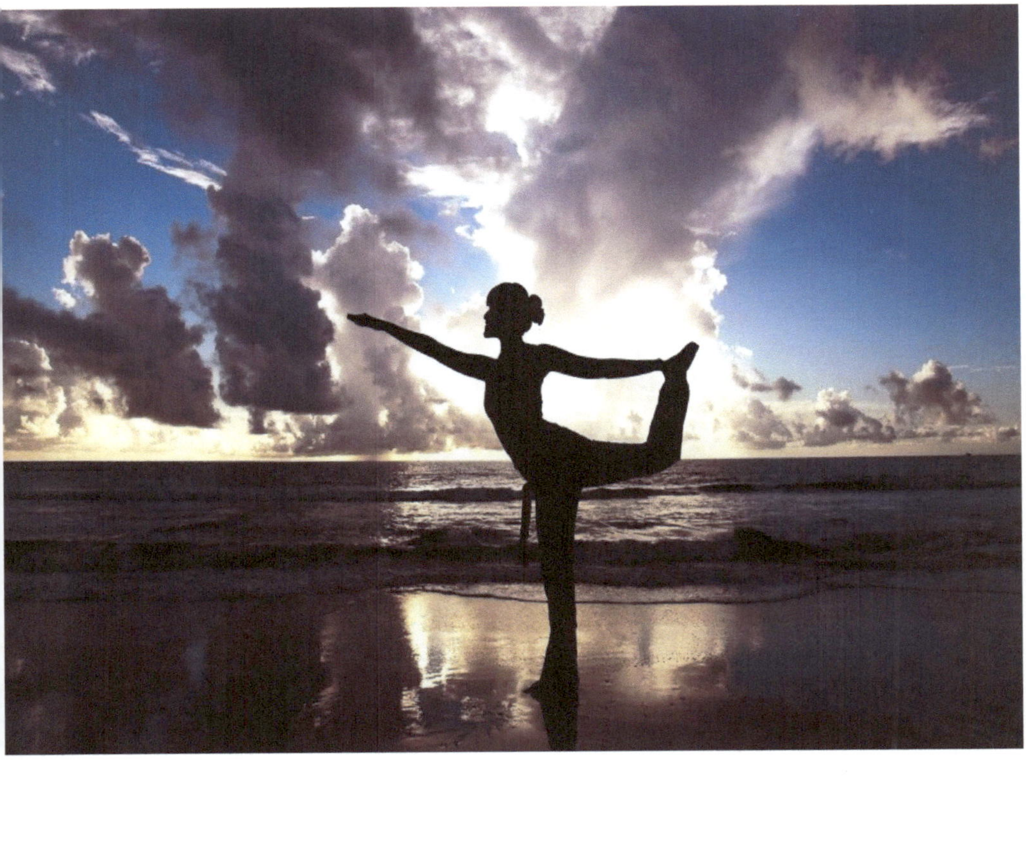

Table of content

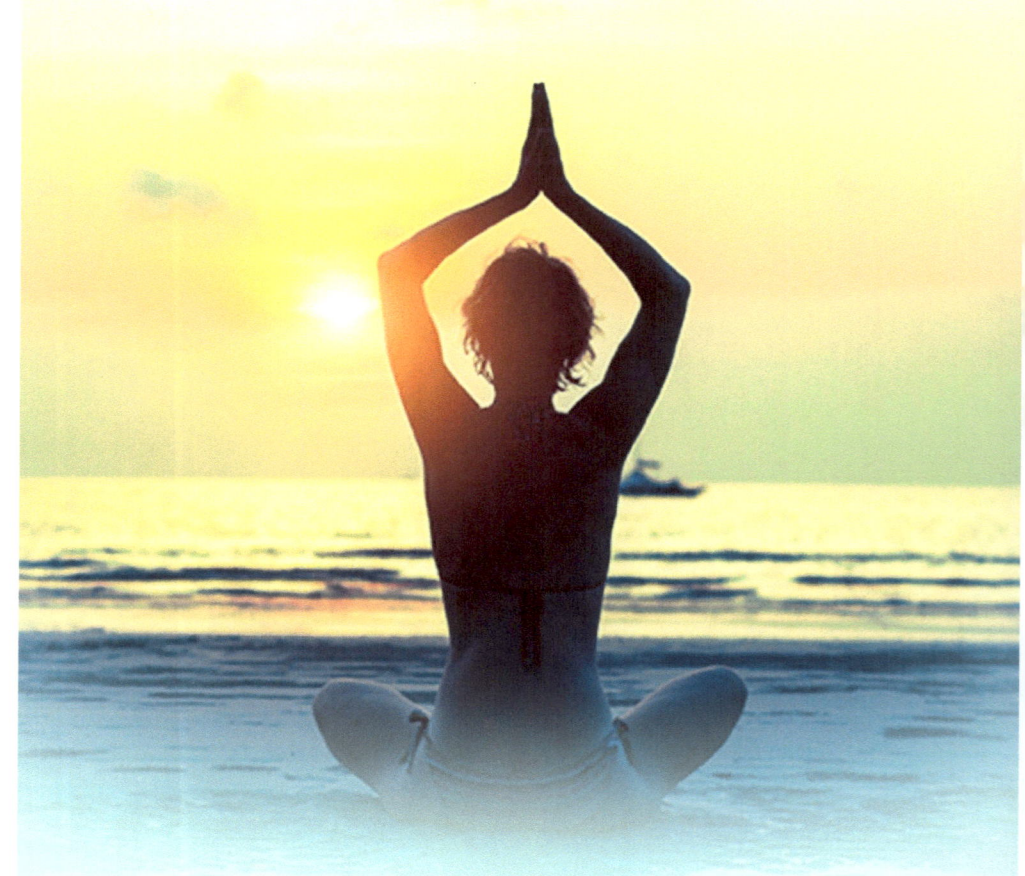

Yoga for Beginners:
THE ULTIMATE YOGA GUIDE FOR NEWBIES

How to Relieve Stress, Lose Weight and find Inner Peace practicing Yoga

Yoga for Beginners: The Ultimate Guide for Newbies.

How to Relieve Stress, Lose Weight and find Inner Peace

By

By Michele Gilbert

<u>Visit My Amazon Author Page</u>

Dedicated to those who choose to stretch beyond their own limits and to seek a more abundant and fulfilling life.

Your thoughts are creative.

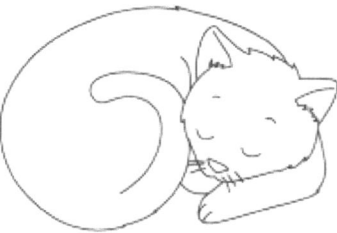

Michele Gilbert

My Free Gift To You!

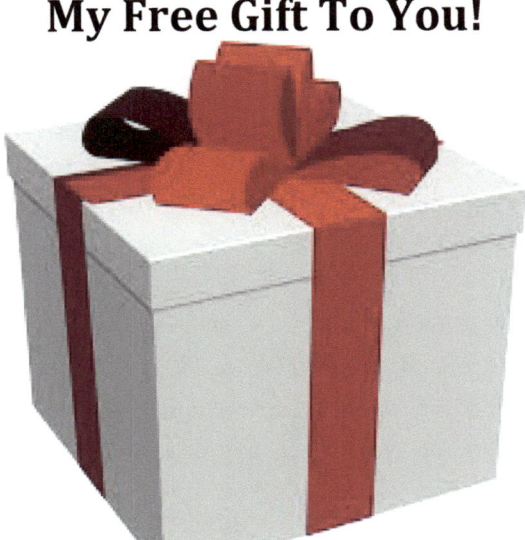

As a way of saying thank you for downloading my book, I am willing to give you access to a selected group of readers who (every week or so) receive inspiring, life-changing kindle books at deep discounts, and sometimes even absolutely free.

Wouldn't it be great to get amazing Kindle offers delivered directly to your inbox?

Wouldn't it be great to be the first to know when I'm releasing new fresh and above all sharply discounted content?

But why would I do something like this?

Why would I offer my books at such a low price and even give them away for free when they took me countless hours to produce?

Simple…. because I want to spread the word!

For a few short days Amazon allows Kindle authors to promote their newly released books by offering them deeply discounted (up to 70% price discounts and even for free. This allows us to spread the word extremely quickly allowing users to download thousands and thousands of copies in a very short period of time.

Once the timeframe has passed, these books will revert back to their normal selling price. That's why you will benefit from being the first to know when they can be downloaded for free!

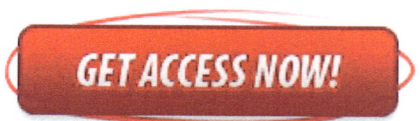

So are you ready to claim your weekly Kindle books?

Introduction

I want to thank you and congratulate you for downloading the book, *"Yoga for Beginners: The Ultimate Guide for Newbies.*

How to Relieve Stress: Lose Weight and find Inner Peace.

This book contains proven steps and strategies on how to practice yoga and achieve your inner peace, live a stress free life and begin to lose weight.

In this book we offer an explanation of the basics of the Yoga technique. By reading the book you will be able to learn how to practice the basics of the technique in order to get the balance back to your body and mind. By following these simple steps you will possibly find a new you. You don`t need any money, a lot of time and effort, you just have to start to live Yoga.

Thanks again for downloading this book, I hope you enjoy it!

What is Yoga?

In the western world it is common to look for a fulfillment outside of ourselves; outer attainments are believed to bring us peace and well being. But, if we take a look back at our own experience we will realize that nothing external can fulfill our longing for something more, something meaningful. The answer to our problems lies in the fact that we have to look deep into ourselves in order to achieve inner peace. The Eastern practices, due to their philosophical background, are based on working on the life conditions from within. One of these practices is the world famous technique of Yoga.

The ancient practice of yoga aims to unify mind, body and spirit. Basically, Yoga is the simple process of reversing the ordinary outward flow of energy in order for mind to become a dynamic center of direct perception, independent of senses. The union between the mind body and spirit can be achieved by different means. One of the ways is meditation, but it is usually necessary to prepare the body for the process by stretching and building physical strength. Many people think that Yoga is just stretching, but the fact is that while stretching you should create the balance in the body through developing strength. There are several basic postures that you will learn in Yoga classes, but some of them will be presented in the book in front of you. In addition to learning postures and exercises, yoga classes can include, and they usually do, instructions on breathing, call and response chanting, meditation, or an inspirational reading of your teacher. There are different ways of teaching Yoga according to the needs of the customers, so whatever you need you will find a suitable class for you.

Yoga for beginners

In this part we will present you some beginner's friendly basic yoga postures that you can try out on your own.

- **Mountain pose**

There are numerous benefits of this pose. It will improve your overall posture and it will improve your sense of center, which is your mind. By practicing this pose regularly you will achieve mental clarity, and also solid breathing.

1) Simply stand, with your feet hip-width apart and parallel. Lift your toes from the ground, spread them and place them back on the floor. You should feel that your weight is evenly balanced; you should not be leaned forwards or backwards.

2) Pull up the knee caps, squeeze the thighs and tuck the tailbone slightly under. Feel that your hips are aligned directly over your ankles. Keep your legs straight.

3) Inhale, and lift out your waist. You should make a movement as pressing your head towards the ceiling in order to stretch your spine.

4) Exhale and lower your shoulders and move them down as you reach the fingertips towards the floor. Slowly press the chest towards the room.

5) Breathe and hold for 5-8 seconds.

There are multiple variations in this pose, most of them regarding the placement of the hands. You can interlace the hands with your index finger pointing up. Also, you can place your arms down with the palms on your outer thighs. Finally, you can place your palms together in front of your heart.

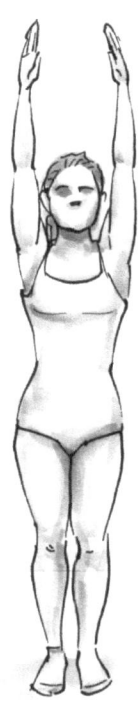

2) Downward facing dog

By practicing this posture you will encourage your full-body circulation, and achieve a great stretch of your calves and heels.

1) Come onto the floor on your hands and knees. Place your knees directly below your hips and your hands slightly forward of your shoulder line. Spread your palms, with your index fingers parallel or slightly turned out. Turn your toes under.

2) Exhale and slowly lift your knees from the ground. At first, your knees should be slightly bent and the heels lifted from the floor. Lengthen your tailbone away from the back of your pelvis and press in lightly towards the pubis. To make a movement against the resistance of your body, in order to keep it effective, lift your sitting bones toward the ceiling and draw the inner legs up into the groins, from your inner ankles.

3) Whilst exhaling, push your top thighs back and stretch your heels onto the floor. Straighten your knees with paying attention not to lock them. Firm the outer thighs and roll the upper thighs slightly inwards. The front of the pelvis should be narrowed.

4) In this step you should firm the outer arms and press your index fingers into the floor. Lift your inner arms from the wrists to the top of your shoulders. Firm your shoulder blades against your back, widen them and draw them toward the tailbone. Keep the head firm between the upper arms.

5) Stay in this pose for 1-3 minutes. Then bend your knees to the floor with exhalation and rest.

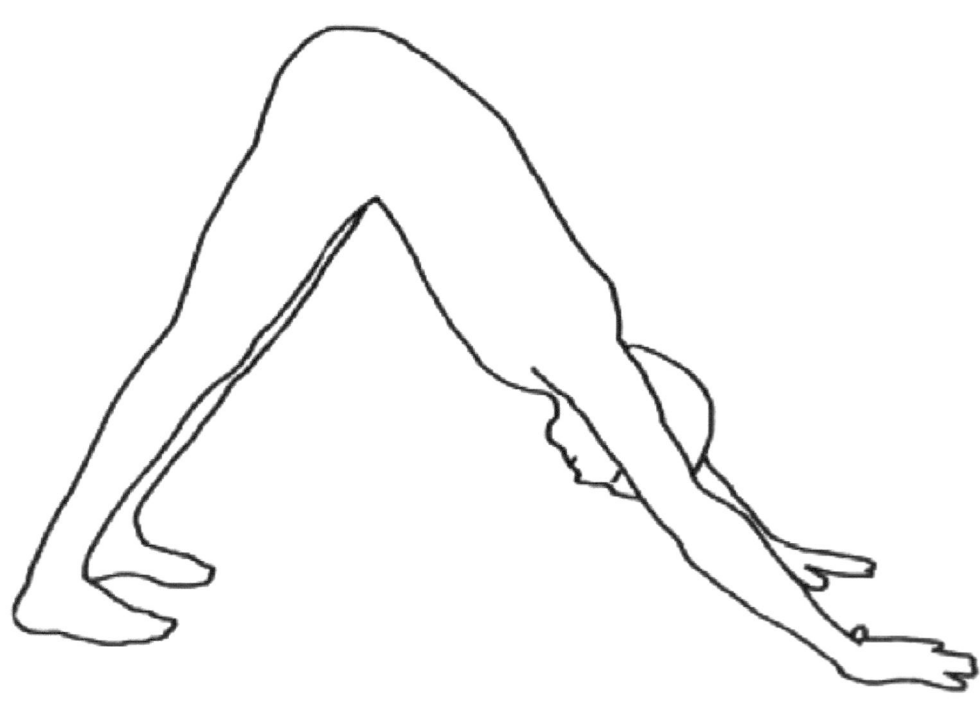

3) Warrior pose

This pose is especially useful for stretching and to strengthen your legs and ankles.

1) Stand in mountain pose. While exhaling, step or lightly jump your feet apart. Raise your arms perpendicular to the floor, keeping them parallel to each other. Reach towards the ceiling. Firm your scapulas against your back and draw them down toward the coccyx.

2) Turn your left foot for 45-60 degrees to the right, and the right one for 90 degrees to the right. Place your right and left heels aligned. Exhale and rotate your torso to the right. As the left hop point turns forward, press the head of the left femur back to ground the heel. Lengthen your coccyx toward the floor, and slightly arch your upper torso.

3) Firmly press your left heel towards the floor. Exhale and bend your right knee over the right ankle, so the shin is perpendicular to the floor. If you feel that you are flexible enough, try and align your right thigh parallel to the floor.

4) Strongly reach through your arms. Lift the ribcage away from the pelvis. As you ground down through the back foot you should feel a lifting sensation running up the back of your legs, across your stomach and chest and up into your arms. If you feel you can do it, bring your palms together. Spread the palms against each other and reach a little higher through the pinky sides of your hands. Your head should be in a neutral position, or tilted back to look up at your thumbs.

5) Stay in this position for 30 seconds to a minute. To finish the exercise you should come up. While coming up, inhale, press the back heel firmly into the floor and reach up through the arms. Turn the feet forward and release the arms while exhaling. Take a few deep breaths, and turn the feet to the left. Slowly return to mountain pose.

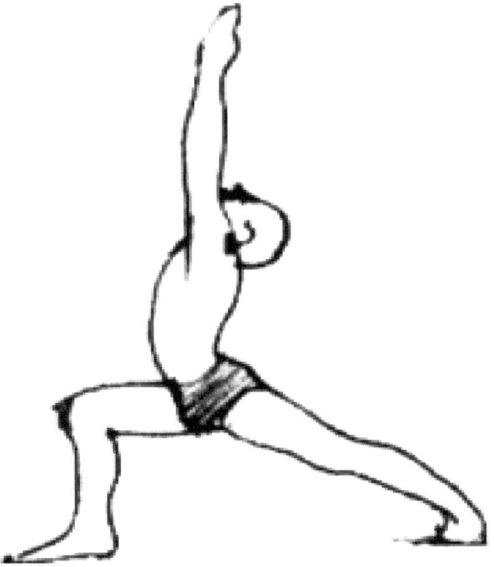

4) Tree pose

With practicing this pose you will improve your balance and strengthen your thighs, calves, ankles and spine.

1) Mountain pose is the basis for this exercise also. So you should stand in mountain pose. Shift your weight to the left foot. While doing this remember to keep the inner foot firm to the floor and bend your right knee. Use your right hand to reach down and if possible clasp your right ankle.

2) Draw your right foot up and place the sole against the inner left thigh. If you feel ready press the right heel into the inner left groin. Toes should be pointed downwards, towards the floor. The center of your pelvis should be placed directly over your left foot.

3) Place your hands on the top rim of your pelvis whilst making sure that the pelvis is in the neutral position, with the top rim parallel to the floor.

4) Lengthen your tailbone toward the floor. Press the foot that is resting on your inner thigh and resist with the outer left leg. Gaze softly at a fixed point in front of you on the floor.

5) Stay in this position for 30 seconds to 1 minute. Return to mountain pose while exhaling and repeat for the same length of time with the other leg.

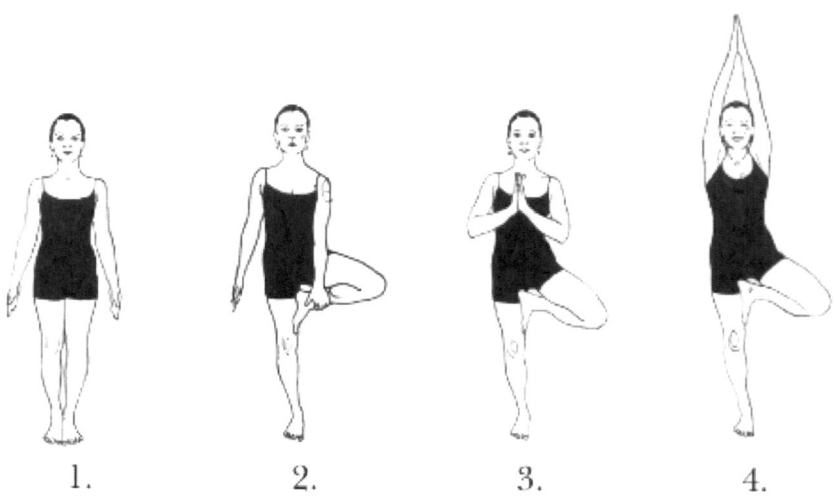

1.   2.   3.   4.

5) Bridge pose

By practicing this posture you will strenghten your chest, neck and spine. You can also use it as a great warm-up for more intense backbends.

) Lie supine on the floor. If you feel the soreness in your shoulders you can place thickly folded blanket or a pillow under them. Bend your knees and place your eet on the floor. Your heels should be as close as possible to your sitting bones.

) Exhale and press your inner feet and arms towards the floor. Push your ailbone upward toward the pubis, firm the buttocks and lift them of the floor owards the ceiling. Keep your thighs and inner feet parallel. Clasp your hands below your pelvis and extend through the arms to help you stay on the tops of our shoulders.

) Lift your buttocks until the thighs are parallel to the floor. Your knees should be over the heels, firmly pressed on the ground. Push them forward, away from the hips. Lift your pubis toward the navel.

) Lift your chin slightly away from the sternum. Firm your shoulder blades and press the top of the sternum toward the chin. Keep your outer arms firmed. Broaden your shoulder blades and try to lift the space between them at the base of your neck, up into the torso.

) Stay in this pose between 30 seconds and 1 minute, as long as you feel comfortable. Adjust the exercise to your physical possibilities. Release with an exhalation.

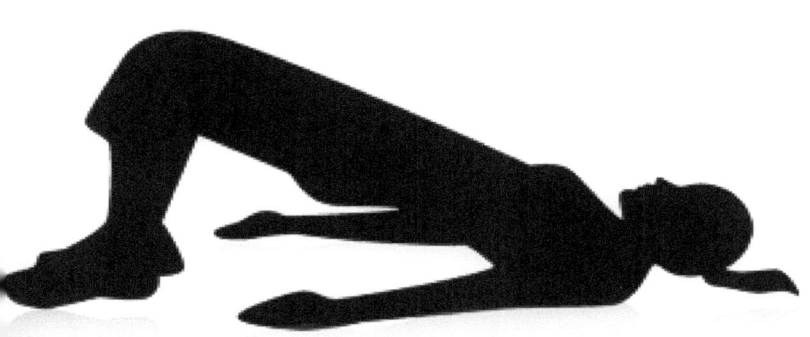

Yoga for weight loss

Yoga is a great way of losing weight if practiced regularly, like any other exercise plan. The advantages of this technique are that it is light on the joints, which is especially useful for over-weight people, and the chances of injuries are minimal. Also, you don`t have to spend thousands of dollars in order to get into an expensive gym program, you can do the exercises from the comfort of your home. Yoga can be combined with other weight loss techniques and exercises.

A lot of celebrities practice Yoga in order to maintain their physical appearance. One of them is Jennifer Aniston, with a body that even younger girls dream about. We will now present you her workout plan in order to help you in your weight loss process. If this program is not suitable for you, you can practice the above described Yoga poses for beginners and you will see the results guaranteed.

1) Temple pose

The target of this exercise is the calves' muscles.

Plant your feet wide and firmly on the ground. Bend your knees out to the side and open at a 90 degree ankle. Sink your butt down in alignment with your knees, squat and hold for 30 minutes. Repeat this movement 8 times. Make a small break and repeat the whole thing. Start with 3 series and move your way up to 7, gradually. Follow the rhythm of your body.

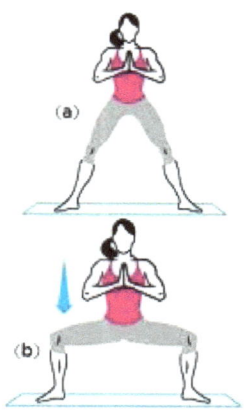

2) Chair pose

The exercise targets legs and buttocks.

Sink down imitating a sinking down in the chair movement. Your feet should be aligned and hip-width apart. In this position move back your weight, from the balls of the feet towards the heels, whilst shifting your hips back. Align your knee over heels with your butt back and peel your belly off your thighs by extending your arms over your head. Do 1-3 sets of this exercise. If you really want to tone up your legs you can combine this exercise with squats.

3) Sun salute

Muscles that are targeted are abs and hamstrings.

Sweep your arms over your head while you are taking a deep breath. As you exhale, dive forward. Place your hands on the floor and extend your chest forward. Step back to the top of a push-up and place your palms directly below your shoulders. Your hips and shoulders should be aligned and then firm your thighs. Lower your body to a push-up and resist the floor. Scoop your chest and arch your body to a position of an upward facing dog and keep your thighs on the floor. Roll over the toes until you get into the position of downward facing dog. Make sure to use your inner thighs and abs whilst doing this movement.

THE SUN
SALUTATION

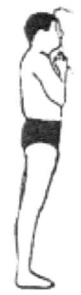

1. exhale

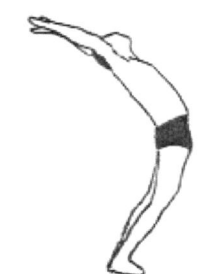

2. inhale

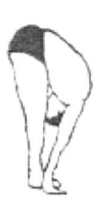

3. exhale

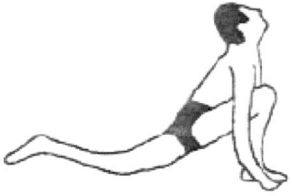

4. inhale

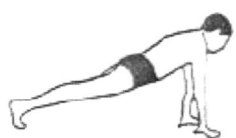

5. retain

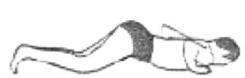

6. exhale

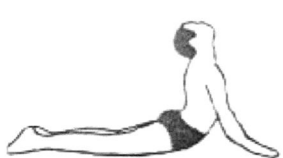

7. inhale

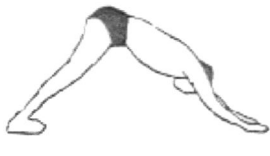

8. exhale

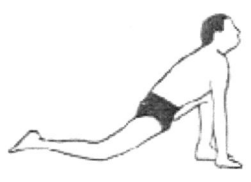

9. inhale

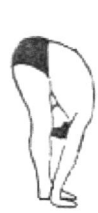

10. exhale

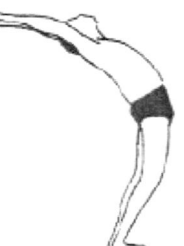

11. inhale

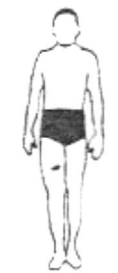

12. exhale,
inhale and begin
again at 1.

4) Reclining Pigeon

The exercise targets chest and thighs.

Lie back with your knees bent and the soles of your feet on the floor. Place your right ankle over your right knee and flex your foot. Move your right knee towards the chest. Wrap around your hamstring and slowly move your knee as near as possible towards your chest. While performing this movement you should feel the stretching of your left hip. Repeat this exercise with your right leg.

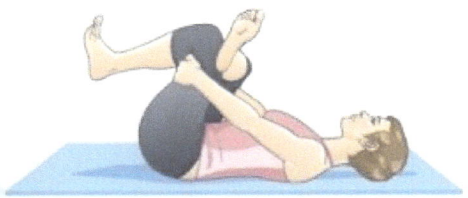

The fifth pose is the tree pose described in the part concerning basic Yoga postures for beginners. In order to achieve the best results, stick to this exercise routine on a daily basis. Keep the positive attitude toward your body and success, it may sound weird but your body recognizes your feelings and reacts to them. The combination of these techniques with meditation, other exercises and positive attitude can lead you to discover new you and to fall in love with yourself.

In order to keep you motivated we will share with you a before and after consistent Yoga practicing photo. Remember, this could be you!

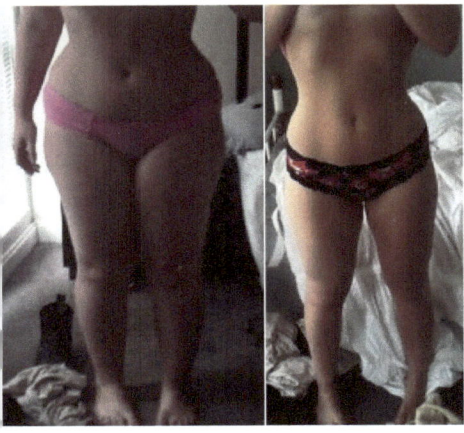

Yoga poses for stress relief

Yoga is known as a stress relief technique, but it can also help you in treating anxiety problems. Yoga is a practice, not a competition. You should not try to move the boundaries of your body and mind, rather, you should focus on what you can easily achieve. It should be a pleasure practicing this famous technique not a pain. In the following part of the book, we will present you the basic sequence of stress relief postures, the steps should be practiced one by one in order to achieve the results. When practicing Yoga in order to achieve inner peace you should focus on your breathing and also free your mind of the worries.

1) Salutation seal

This pose is practiced in order to achieve a meditative state of awareness. Your palms should be placed against each other in front of your heart. This way of placing your hands represents the unification of the right and left side of your body. You should sit in a cross legged position with your eyes closed. By taking this position you prepare yourself for meditation.

2) Easy pose

This pose will help you achieve the inner calm. You should retain the sitting position with your hips wide open and a straight spine. But place your hands on your knees and rest for at least 60 seconds. Focus on your breathing.

3) Cat pose

This pose will massage your spine and belly organs, while, at the same time, it helps you beat the stress. Place your knees on the ground and your hands also. Your back should be arched and your head down. Your wrists should be directly under your shoulder, and knees under the hips. Stay in this pose for 2 minutes, while breathing evenly. This pose will also help you stimulate the digestive tract.

4) Cow pose

From the previous cat pose, you should lower your back and lift your head up. The wrists and knees should stay in the same alignment as in the previous pose. This pose, as the cat pose will have same physical benefits, but it will also help you calm your mind.

5) Child`s pose

You should now place your thighs on your calves and your belly on your thighs and extend your arms over your head. Your forehead should be rested on the ground. You can make alterations to this pose, as with any other to chose the posture that best suits your needs.

After finishing these postures, which are a part of one sequence, you can return to the salutation seal in order to finish the cycle. Try to completely free your mind and feel the peace that is overwhelming you. Focus on deep breathing and then open your eyes.

These exercises won`t take you a lot of time and you can do them when you wake up, or right before you go to the bed. You should just stick to the routine. It will make you feel great. If you want to achieve the best results, you can combine weight loss and stress relief techniques, it would then be the whole package.

Yoga diet plan

As with any other technique, the physical exercise should be followed by a proper diet. This is not a food plan made only for those who want to lose weight, it is made for everybody who wants to live healthy and practice Yoga to the fullest.

Many yoga diets are pure vegetarian, but even if you include fish and meat, the basis should be vegetables. Other foods that should be included in your regular nutrition plan are fruits, whole grains, seeds, nuts and legumes, such as beans and lentils. Food that grows in the sun has the most valued properties in Yoga dieting.

How you prepare your food and eat it is equally important as what you eat. Prepare and eat your meals with love and awareness. Also, you should not eat 2-3 hours before the practicing of Yoga. Still if you have to, the best solution is bananas, oatmeal, pears, apples, rice, low-fat yoghurt or veggies.

Start changing your life today and enjoy the journey!

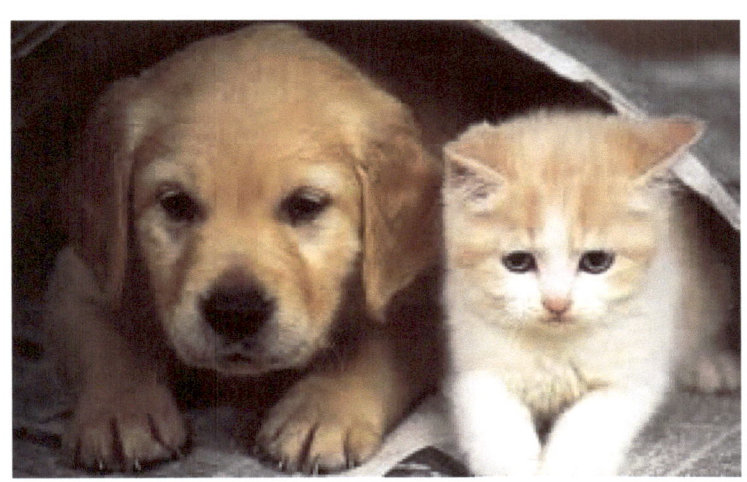

Before you go, I'd like to say thank you for purchasing my book.

I know you could have picked so many other books to read .But you took a chance on me.

So A Big thanks for downloading this book and reading it all the way to completion.

Now I would like to ask a _small_ favor.

Could you please take a minute or two to leave a review for this book on Amazon?

<u>Click here</u>

The feedback will help me continue to publish more kindle books that will help people to get better results in their lives.

And if you found it helpful in anyway then please let me know :-)

Preview of My New Book

WICCA

THE ULTIMATE BEGINNERS GUIDE FOR WITCHES AND WARLOCKS

LEARN WICCA MAGIC SPELLS, TRADITIONS AND RITUALS

MICHELE GILBERT

What is Wicca?

So you're interested in Wicca, or maybe you've already started your adventure into the big world of one of the oldest religions in the world. It's a noble quest, as is the pursuit of higher knowledge in any religion. For you to continue your journey, or perhaps to start it, you're going to need to begin somewhere and reading is always the best place to start. So here you go.

To be honest, Wicca has, like every religion, evolved over the long years that it has existed. What started as blind paganism and mysticism has adapted and evolved, tearing apart the cruel ambition, dark rituals, and bloody rites that gave it a sense of barbarism. What is left is the enlightened, adapted version of the old ways that have been passed down for ages. Like most religions, there are sects and factions, all of which have ideological differences that distinguish them. But for a brief history on the faith, I will be your esteemed guide through history.

Let's start at the beginning:

In the early twentieth century, the idea of Wicca was first born. Yes, we do trace our roots all the way back to the foundations of religion itself and it is often said that we are one of the oldest faiths because of this. However, to be quite honest, so do most religions. Wicca itself was founded by the meeting of clandestine groups that some call covens. Wait, let me clarify, we call them covens. Our faith existed in silence and in secrecy due to Christian persecution. Originating mostly from European traditions and resurgence in the mystic arts, it wasn't until the Fifties that we were actually given the name the Craft. This was really the capitalistic boom of our religion, which, from my own personal beliefs, is one of our darker periods. We were much more interested in popularity and attention rather than the pursuit of the Craft.

What you are stepping into now is a much different faith than was previously established in the Sixties and the Seventies after the sensational blossom of our beliefs in the Fifties took root. Today, most Wicca practitioners that you meet are quietly dedicated to the faith and beliefs that they have been taught. Though there are many covens in the world today, meeting and practicing, it is a deeply personalized faith that we follow and it is dedicated to a lot of independent research and development.

Here's what we do not do, or at least to the best of my knowledge. We do not eat babies, we do not worship the devil, and we do not offer human sacrifices. Like I have said before, our faith is extremely popularized by society, no thanks to some of our own members.

Honestly, if you were to meet an average Wiccan on the streets, you probably wouldn't know it. Sure, we draw an element of society, the lost souls, the searching, and the misunderstood. We welcome them and we give them a community, but we're good people and we are not all witches or warlocks.

But, on the other hand, we do practice magic. Yes, I said it. The elephant in the room has been addressed. That's why you're here after all? Isn't that the lure of the Wiccan faith? Magic? The fact that we acknowledge and believe what everyone in their heart secretly knows that the elements and the forces of the physical and spiritual world are very real and present. Sure, we dabble with primordial forces, but with respect and understanding. No, I cannot turn you into a cat and no I cannot kill you with a spell.

Any true Wicca would rather die than use magic improperly, because there is always a price when it comes to magic.

So, have I piqued your curiosity? Are you interested in knowing more? Then come on in and don't be shy. We'll have a nice little chat and you'll see what it really means to be a Wiccan and I'll tell you about the magic that you know in your heart to be real. I'll give a glimpse at the other side of the world, beyond cell phones and the Internet, where the forests loom and the shadows lurk. There are forces beyond all of us and if you want to know more, I will gladly be your guide.

Concerning Covens:

If you are taking the path that leads you to becoming a Wiccan, you're not like everyone else. You're special, because we do not have Churches, Mosques, or Synagogues on every corner. You will not find temples or university groups, well, you might find a university group or two, but not many. There are a lot of people who like to put on makeup and dress funny and claim to be Wiccans, which makes it hard for newcomers to find a home. If you're serious about becoming a Wiccan or delving into any of the neopagan groups, there are many resources.

Thankfully, we've evolved as a people and the Internet has become a wonderful way for us to connect. After all, Wiccans make up less than one percent of the religious community in America, which makes it hard for our brothers and sisters in Nowhere, Nebraska to commune with us. Thanks to the Internet, there's now a way for us to communicate and encourage one another. It's truly a great tool for us to use.

To read the rest click below!

Wicca: The Ultimate Beginners Guide For Witches and Warlocks: Learn Wicca Magic Spells, Traditions and Rituals

P.S. You'll find many more books like this and others under my name Michele Gilbert.

Don't miss them… here is a short list.

Introduction To Palmistry: The Ultimate Palm Reading Guide For Beginners

Emotional Intelligence: How to Succeed By Mastering Your Emotions And Raising Your IQ

Wicca: The Ultimate Beginners Guide For Witches and Warlocks: Learn Wicca Magic

The Introvert's Advantage: The Introverts Guide To Succeeding In An Extrovert World

Stop Playing Mind Games: How To Free Yourself Of Controlling And Manipulating Relationships

Instant Charisma: A Quick And Easy Guide To Talk, Impress, And Make Anyone Like You

Chakras: Understanding The 7 Main Chakras For Beginners: The Ultimate Guide To Chakra Mindfulness, Balance and Healing

Practicing Mindfulness: Living in the moment through Meditation: Everyday Habits and Rituals to help you achieve inner peace

Adrenal Fatigue: What Is Adrenal Fatigue Syndrome And How To Reset Your Diet And Your Life

Body Language 101: What A Person's Body Language Is Really Telling You...And How You Can Use It To Your Advantage

Sleep Tight: Overcome Insomnia and Sleep Disorders for a better more restful sleep!

The Arthritis Pain Cure: How to find Arthritis Pain Relief and live a happy pain free life!

The Headache Pain Cure: How to find Headache Pain Relief and live a happy Pain Free Life!

Stop Panic Attacks and Anxiety Disorders without Drugs Now!: Overcome Panic, Stress and Anxiety and live a happy pain free life!

The Breakup Recovery Guide: Advice for Surviving Heartbreak, Letting Go and Thriving in an exciting new life!

The Friendship Guide to Finding Friends Forever: How to Find, Make and Keep Quality Friendships After your Breakup

The Credit Fix: Leave behind credit card debt and poor credit scores and get your life back!

How To Stop Being Jealous And Insecure: Overcome Insecurity And Relationship Jealousy

My Free Gift To You!

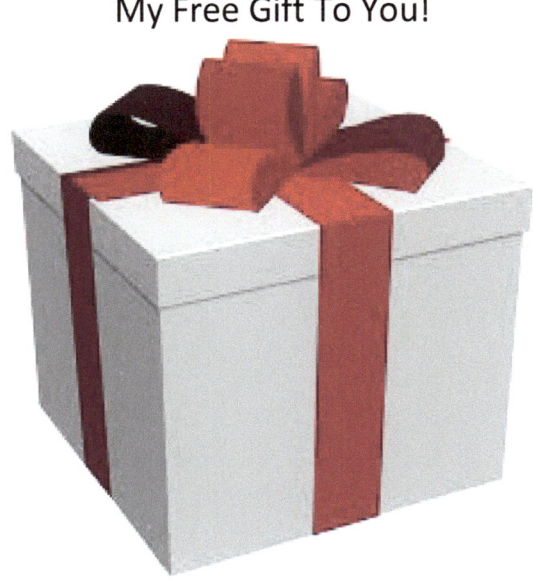

As a way of saying thank you for downloading my book, I am willing to give you access to a selected group of readers who (every week or so) receive inspiring, life-changing kindle books at deep discounts, and sometimes even absolutely free.

Wouldn't it be great to get amazing Kindle offers delivered directly to your inbox?

Wouldn't it be great to be the first to know when I'm releasing new fresh and above all sharply discounted content?

But why would I do something like this?

Why would I offer my books at such a low price and even give them away for free when they took me countless hours to produce?

Simple…. because I want to spread the word.!

For a few short days Amazon allows Kindle authors to promote their newly released books by offering them deeply discounted (up to 70% price discounts and even for free. This allows us to spread the word extremely quickly allowing users to download thousands and thousands of copies in a very short period of time.

Once the timeframe has passed, these books will revert back to their normal selling price. That's why you will benefit from being the first to know when they can be downloaded for free!

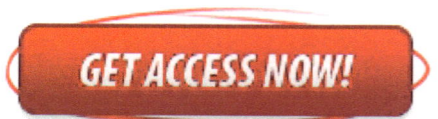

So are you ready to claim your weekly Kindle books?

You are just one click away! Follow the link below and sign up to start receiving awesome content

Thank you and Enjoy!

About Michele

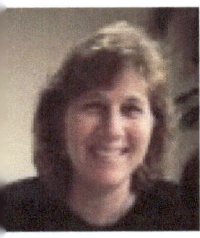

Michele Gilbert was born and raised in Brooklyn, New York. Drawn to literature and writing at a young age, she enrolled at Brooklyn College and majored in English. After graduation Michele did not begin writing immediately, instead she embarked on a career in the finance industry and spent the next thirty years on Wall Street.

Serendipity struck when she least expected it. After ending a long-term relationship, Michele found herself lost and unsure what the future held. She began to read books on grief and loss, looking for answers. Those led her to delve deeper into the Law of Attraction and its power. What resulted was remarkable. Not only had she begun to heal, she had also rekindled her former love of writing and discovered her life's purpose.

The years have taken her through many twists and turns, but she learned valuable lessons along the way. Today she publishes books-mostly self-help and metaphysical in nature-and feels compelled to share her knowledge with those facing similar experiences. Her greatest hope is to inspire others and show them ways to overcome adversity and gracefully accept life's inevitable low points.

Going forward, she plans to incorporate more teachings of self-help, finance and meditation. Regular meditation is very beneficial to her progress as she forges a new life. Morning rituals and positive incantations are other practices Michele embraces; they are very restorative in daily life.

As an avid hiker, Michele and fellow club members often hike the picturesque Jersey Pine Barrens. She is a history buff, voracious reader, baseball fanatic and a foodie. She also proudly supports Trout Unlimited-a national non-profit organization dedicated to conserving, protecting and restoring North America's Coldwater fisheries and their watersheds.

Michele currently resides forty minutes from Atlantic City and the Jersey Shore. She makes her home with a Blue Russian rescue cat named Jersey, though she isn't exactly sure who rescued who.

Michele really enjoys publishing books that can make a difference in people's lives. If you have any suggestions or would like to have a specific topic covered in a future book, please send an email to michelegilbertbooks@gmail.com and we will get back to you.

Thanks for reading!